MW00644133

Dearest
Karen,

Over the many
years We have shared
some good music,
laughter + come to truth
moments... It's been a
pleasure having you as a
client/friend. Blessings
Thank U for your
continued support—
XOXO

LESIA M. DAVIS

TAKING THE BEAST OUT OF BEAUTY

a **COLLECTION** *of* **HAIR CARE SECRETS**

from **34 YEARS** *of* **EXPERIENCE**

CONTENTS

FOREWORD 1
   Simplicity Isn't Easy... 1

SHAMPOOING 3
   Shampoo: 4
   Filters: 4
   Dry Shampoo: 6
   CoWash: 7
   Color Enhancing Shampoo: 8
   pH: Potential Hydrogen 8
   Botanicals: 9
   Saturation: 11
   Frequency: 14

CONDITIONING 16
   Is This Really Necessary? 16
   Supple Application: 20
   The Spiral: 21
   Detangling: 22
   Stress-less Hair: 23

DETANGLING AGAIN 35
   Implements: 37

FINISHING 39
   Flat Iron: 43

BRUSHING 44

VITAMINS, NUTRITION, and ESSENTIAL OILS ... 48

PSYCHOLOGY 53

ACKNOWLEDGMENTS 55

RESOURCES 57

FOREWORD

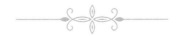

Long Hair Goals-
Healthy Hair-
Treat your hair as you'd treat your skin!
(Just imagine what would happen!)-
Hair Harmony and You-

Simplicity Isn't Easy...

I use these phrases often because of the many people I encounter; many absolutely hate their hair. Once I realized my super thick hair had started thinning from all the tactics I'd use to transform it into something it wasn't, I had an epiphany: STOP and LOVE on your hair!

Hair has been my obsession since I was four years young, from styling my grandmother's wigs on Sundays to cutting my doll's hair and then onto live bait—my family. It was my medium for creating textures and experimenting with products designated for certain hair and skin types. I saw beyond the skin tone; I just saw universal texture. I focused on creating solutions for what seemed like the impossible.

The possibilities were endless. I had a vision and I wanted to conquer the world!

Since beginning my career I have had the fortune of experimenting on and practicing with my clients, who have taken me to Vienna, Rome, Miami, New York, DC, and places in between.

It has been an incredible journey that has allowed me to incorporate all of my experiences to enhance my application to hair along the way.

This handbook is meant to reveal how these simple techniques toward grooming, restoring, and transforming your hair and body can give you the beautiful head of hair you were intended to have with the hair texture you are blessed with.

Once you have made peace with your hair and have improved your habits, with some patience you will truly be surprised at how simple healthy hair can be...

SHAMPOOING

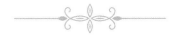

Water, shampoo, CoWash, or dry shampoo? The first step…

My clients frequently ask how often they need to shampoo. Do weekly suds and water dry out the hair? How frequently should they clarify? Is a shampoo for color-treated hair necessary?

How efficient is dry shampoo, or is a CoWash technique best?

What I am about to share with you is what I have experienced in the 30-plus years of my restoring and growing hair that will complement your existing hair care routine.

I will share some tips that will help your wellness regimen and some valuable techniques that are conducive for effective cleansing.

These are simple, tried, and true remedies that will become part of your lifestyle.

My first suggestion is that, in order for your hair to look and feel its absolute best, shampoo as often as you feel it is necessary to remove environmental pollutants.

This is the first step toward a cleansed scalp, which is crucial to the foundation of healthy hair!

One essential component is oxygen. Cleansing creates a healthy environment for the skin and supports air flow, which enables the hair to grow and thrive.

Shampoo:

In keeping with the flow, cleansing with fresh water and a liquid or a cream shampoo is my preferred combination for purification and feeling renewed. Without question water cleanses most effectively, removing and rinsing away buildup of product and sluggish skin and irritants that inhibit the hair from flowing. In my opinion this is the beginning for luminous, youthful-looking hair full of life and body.

Filters:

Another component for creating a beautiful crown is using filtered water if possible.

Imagine using pure, clean water flowing from a spring and rinsing your hair with it … refreshing, huh?

Cleansing and rinsing your hair using filtered aqua, thus removing the negative ions from this resource, fulfills that imaginative experience and the benefits are amazing.

The water is softer; it reduces chlorine and captures the additives that can dry the skin and hair.

As a result, your hair is shinier, your strands remain hydrated, and your tinted hair lasts much longer!

Getting and using filter water can be achieved in a few ways.

One is by using a home water filtration system. If this isn't feasible, then a portable filter on your showerhead is easily attainable and more budget friendly. The device will capture minute particles and chemicals that can impede the hair from receiving the optimum benefits from your hair care products. Another component to using the purest water possible is to clean your showerhead. Simply disassemble the showerhead and soak it in a calcium cleanser and it will remove any build up that has settled in the showerhead. The final step to this technique is to run the water through the showerhead before using again.

A final alternative is boiling your water. This ancient method has been used for centuries, removing impurities and purifying this valuable resource.

However, CAUTION!

Allow ample time for the boiling water to cool before using. If this last technique sounds arduous and like too much work for your repeated shampoos, then perhaps save the prepared aqua for your last and final rinse. Something tried is better than nothing at all.

This boiling method was my daily routine for removing particles for my family and I before bottled water became the precautionary standard for consumption. Regularly, while preparing the water for my morning tea, I simply poured the extra liquid into a glass container after it had settled from the day. Then the next morning I started refilling my kettle anew.

This sounds like a lot of work, but it actually becomes effortless. This ritual is also a cost saver. It saves money on bottled water for drinking. It is great also for your houseplants, especially re-blooming orchids!

Okay, returning to hair.

Once again, the benefit that comes with using filtered water is that your hair is devoid of unsuspecting traces of minerals and calcium that come from even your natural surroundings.

These undetected harsh sediments can be the source of the hair's baffling brittleness and mysterious dryness that subsequently contribute to continuous breakage and split ends.

When it is possible to use these devices, or alternative methods your hair and scalp will thank you, and you will discover one single element toward Taking the Beast out of Beauty!

Carry on—let's explore and determine which cleansing method is best suited for you to enhance your hair care routine. Let's continue with the variety of shampoos and the latest trends and techniques and their benefits.

Dry Shampoo:

Get gorgeous in an instant!
Why would one use a dry shampoo?

A dry shampoo will lift flat hair at the scalp and is a great way to refresh your hair when you are in a crunch, when time won't allow for soap and water. This process is also designed to remove excess oil and product from the scalp, proving more volume for hair that has been flattened by sebum, which are natural oils produced from the sebaceous glands.

A dry shampoo is a great tool that also gives hair texture, supporting a creative haircut and a definitive style like the '70s shag that has seen a resurgence.

The clay powder or spray is a bodybuilding foundation for molding an updo, or a topknot or piecing and defining a short haircut when water won't do.

Another reason to try dry shampoo is that it's a great alternative to use when conserving water.

In times of drought in respective regions, or when acknowledging environmental change and the need to preserve essential and limited natural resources, dry shampoo can play an integral part in conserving water.

Traveling light, especially these days …

Grab your dry shampoo brand of choice and go.

When you need a refresher, voilà! There's dry shampoo!

I always highly suggest following manufacturers' instructions for optimum results. They have done the research…

CoWash:

Another option for refreshing your crown is the CoWash, a popular cleansing technique opposed to the traditional method of shampooing with a cleanser that produces suds. The CoWash method is popular amongst naturalists seeking an alternative sulfate-free cleansing process. This method involves using a conditioner to cleanse in lieu of a shampoo and is intended to address concerns that come with dehydrating the hair strands as done with traditional cleansing.

This practice is growing and becoming most popular with people who have curly or dry hair, or who adorn braids and locks for hairstyles. Again, in lieu of shampoo, this method substitutes cleanser for a conditioner and rinses with water to remove environmental pollutants from the hair. Using this method, the cuticle remains flat. Conditioner doesn't open the shaft; instead the conditioner seeps into the shaft and releases unwanted pollutants. The results are that the hair feels less coarse and maintains a defined texture or curl pattern.

Color Enhancing Shampoo:

Addressing the question about formulated shampoos for tinted hair. "Are they better?"

Yes, they are, formulated with ingredients that prevent fading and oxidation, accentuating the brilliance of the hue. These shampoos are designed to enhance your color while maintaining a healthy pH balance. By buffering the cuticle, the hair retains moisture, vibrancy and reflects light! Whichever your method of choice, water is the most potent and effective agent to remove impurities and pollutants from most anything. Never underestimate the power of a relaxing shampoo as it is another step toward taking the Beast out of Beauty!

pH: Potential Hydrogen

Having a better understanding of where you stand brings about better choices.

Let's take a look at the balance of the pH scale—neutral, acidic, or alkaline. A healthy pH level for the hair is the range between five and seven. The number seven in this case stands for neutral on the pH scale for skin and hair. The numbers from 0 to 6.9 are on the acidic side, and products ranging from 3.0 to 6.9 are formulated to keep the imbrications closed and maintain their structure.

So, when hair has a propensity for dryness, be cognizant in selecting products in this range, which keep the scales of the cuticle tight and are in general labeled for dry hair. pH numbers from 8 to 14 fall on the alkaline side of the scale, and products in this range are more effective with oily hair types.

On the flip side of dry, if your hair's imbrications are already flat, you may appreciate a product starting, between 7.1 and 9, raising the cuticle slightly and managing excessive sebum and impure scalps. This is a tiny bit of general knowledge to keep in mind when choosing a cleansing system. Neutral is a safe place to be in order to ensure a healthy balance for the epidermis and your strands. When and where there are any major medical concerns, the best advice is to consult a dermatologist.

In today's ever-changing world with more botanical, clean, pure, safe, green, and even vegan shampoo to choose from, it is hard to keep up. However, we are better informed, to make choices.

Botanicals:

Arriving back at the genesis, choosing nature, enriching our lives with botanicals and minerals, and understanding the science of it all helps us thrive in our beauty.

Botanicals like avocado, almond, argan, and sunflower from nature's bounty, infused to hydrate and calm our hair concerns with healing balms, are on the acidic side of the scale.

Rose extracts soften and detangle the hair, soothing tender scalps, especially for children, who tend to have an abundant amount of hair.

We seek naturally derived products in order to provide slip and manageability for the hair and to create a pleasurable hair care experience. Alkaline purifiers address impure scalps prone to psoriasis, dandruff, and dermatological conditions. Kaolin, menthol, marigold, and yarrow, which all are anti-inflammatory botanicals, calm the scalp without compromising dryness, combating recurring flakes and addressing forms of mild fungus that may occur when the hair is consistently damp.

For those looking for prescribed cleansers that yield results and that are formulated with a concentration of healing botanicals specifically for individual needs, these gems can be found in salons, spas, cosmetic emporiums and health stores. The beauty industry is realizing consumers are seeking holistic remedies that are milder and gentler, conforming to a healthier lifestyle without synthetics.

The shampoo need not be harsh, it is the simplest ingredient toward maintaining healthy hair. With the array of products to sample and choose from, lets go through the technique on how to manually shampoo for optimum results!

Saturation:

The first step, rinsing the hair thoroughly before applying shampoo, is the gateway to paradise.

Before applying the first drop of shampoo, saturate your hair thoroughly, relying on the pressure from the water to loosen debris, oils, hair products, dandruff, soot, and all other pollutants that attach themselves to the hair and scalp.

Not only does this feel oh soooo gooood, it also increases blood flow, stimulating the scalp!

Blood flow is actual food for the scalp, producing thicker hair growth. (More on this in the nutrition chapter.) I suggest the best place to cleanse the hair is in the shower, where there is plenty of free-flowing water, as if you were in the salon.

Shampooing in the shower is much better than leaning over a sink hoping for a thorough rinse. The shower is the best place to prevent ill rinsing, and it allows the hair to flow in one direction, preventing snarls and tangles. Remember, as I mentioned before, if you have only one shot for filtered water, let it be your last rinse.

One of my favorite shampoos is Barex's NutriRich Shampoo with Brazil & Macadamia Nut.

It delicately removes impurities from the hair while providing the essential ingredients for nourishing the scalp. It is an essential ingredient in my arsenal of tools, which I use as part of the growing process I am known for. Begin with squeezing a dollop of shampoo into your hands and applying it to your scalp, while separating the hair into sections.

Short hair needs two sections and long hair needs about four sections; this will allow the shampoo to get directly onto the scalp inside the hair and along the length, while distributing the cleanser equally between the strands, producing lather and removing soil and dead skin that clogs the pores.

Next, massage the scalp moderately—be mindful not to crumble the hair into your hands while continuing to knead or massage the shampoo down the length of the hair clear to the ends.

This delicate application prevents bunching and roughing the hair into a ball, tangling and ultimately raising the cuticle. Practice applying this technique for all hair types and lengths. This application will amplify your end results.

The hair ultimately will be smoother and silkier because the hair's imbrications (protective layer) aren't compromised, leaving the cuticle intact. Take into account that the first shampoo exfoliates and loosens pollutants, oils, and flakes from the scalp. Be mindful there isn't a lot of lather from the initial shampoo.

Starting with the first shampoo (especially if you are using a sulfate-free product), continue to shampoo for at least two minutes. The shampoo contains restorative ingredients, so be patient and don't rush through this process. Repeat this step for your second shampoo. Repeat the first step, and the shampoo will glide and slip through the entire head of hair much easier. Continue for at least another two to three minutes, massaging from the scalp, again gently kneading to the ends.

Another note about long hair: you may need to apply just a bit more shampoo to the shaft to ensure the length of the hair hasn't been neglected. Avoiding the ends also results in tangling, split ends, and compromised length (unwanted short hair).

TIP: Don't forget about the hairline (aka the edges), the front of the nape, and behind the ears where hair gathers. This area requires special attention and is often neglected during the cleansing and conditioning process.

I like to apply a little extra attention to and around these areas, which are often either scrubbed too harshly or avoided altogether. Often under-rinsing also leaves residue. This is the catalyst for the beginning stage of flakes and breakage. Water, helps calm an irritated epidermis, soothing the scalp, reversing inflammation, and healing distressed hair. As you begin cleansing your hair, follow the manufacturers' suggestions; you will get the best results from your product.

My last step in the shampoo process is to rinse well with water; removing all traces of the shampoo, rinse until the water runs clear. If you're leaving any lingering residue in the hair it can hinder its flow to grow. Remember the skin must breathe to survive, and exfoliating dead cells produces a healthy, glowing scalp!

Shampooing properly stimulates blood flow, nourishing the papilla and producing healthy follicles and thicker, shinier hair. Another good habit is to shampoo wigs, brushes and combs, sweat bands, hair ties, and all hair accessories when you shampoo your hair. (To extend your wigs' longevity use these same techniques.) Keep your accessories in rotation, and you will never be caught in a pinch!

Remember to include scarfs and bonnets as well!

This is another step toward prevention of hair loss, especially around the hairline, where perspiration, makeup, and oils can settle into the fabric.

Frequency:

Another frequently asked question is: Can I skip the shampoo?

My experience has taught me that a fresh head of hair is the best way to stay ready!

If you feel your weekly shampoo is too frequent, stall only for a short while longer… Like anything dingy, unwashed hair will continue to attract more dirt, which then compromises the integrity of the scalp's airflow, which can lead to unseasoned shedding.

If your natural texture tends toward the dry end of the spectrum, then perhaps less frequently works in your favor. Perhaps one shampoo is better than two. Here also is where the CoWash method may work for you.

Everyone's barometer is different; your dry hair isn't someone else's dryness.

Another point of concern if you notice a lingering sour scent in your hair, take precautions. Chances are fungus may have started to manifest in the hair and on the scalp.

If you work out daily and you take a shortcut with your hair, wearing a wet bun repeatedly, the opportunity for fungus is ripe.

A shampoo with menthol or peppermint may reverse the aggression in the hair or on the scalp.

If there is real cause for concern, don't hesitate to see your dermatologist. Other candidates for fungus are ardent swimmers and bun and ponytail wearers. Those who wear extensions, wigs, or weaves 90 percent of the time need to take precautions and ensure air flow, drying the hair and scalp completely to prevent irreversible hair loss.

Set ample time aside for your hair care routine. The results will be much more gratifying than when you are in a hurry. Those beautiful selfies are well worth it!

Love on your hair...

CONDITIONING

Is This Really Necessary?

Yes, it is beneficial beyond belief!

Another timeless question is, "Can I skip the conditioning process?" I would prefer you didn't… Conditioning the hair has a significant influence on reviving the quality and improvement of your tresses. Once the shampoo process is completed, this is the perfect time to prepare your hair for deeper love in the nourishing department.

However, there is always an exception to the rule.

If the hair tends to lean toward the oily side, resulting in flat, lifeless hair, you, my friend, may consider conditioning every now and again. Your oily scalp serves you well as a natural conditioner, and it is a blessing in disguise. Formulated treatments are available to enhance and balance all hair types.

A burdock-infused remedy is one such treatment. Burdock's anti-sebum properties are used to restore the natural balance of the scalp without weighing it down. Throughout the years, I've witnessed the benefit of natural oil, aid in accelerated hair growth, as the sebum from the scalp glides down the length of the hair shaft and provides natural protection from stress.

On the other hand, if your scalp produces a minimum amount of sebum, or the sebum gets trapped in the pockets of the curl, enabling the oil to glide down the shaft tends to reflect dryness. This is where infusing moisture or conditioner with amino acids comes in to enhance hydration and strength. Compare conditioning your hair with exercising the body for vigor and vitality. Your hair responds in the same manner to a conditioner. It only gets better and better!

Continuing with the hair restorative process…

Once you have rinsed the hair thoroughly, use a towel or a washcloth to squeeze the excess water from your hair, thus removing the barrier that inhibits maximum absorption of nutrients into the hair. This step allows the product the ability to penetrate the cuticle, deepening the nourishing process that facilitates the hairs restoration and boosts its health and luster. Be mindful to caress your tresses, kneading the conditioner smoothly, moving your fingers or a large comb in one direction. Important, focus particularly on the ends, remembering to keep your hair tangle free as much as possible without bunching or crunching your strands, protecting the length.

Finding a conditioner that best fits your particular needs…

For porous or coarse hair, generally speaking, moisture is the best place to start to impart hydration and soften and smooth your strands. Here are few ingredients to consider, used medicinally for centuries to heal and nourish.

Botanicals continued…

Indigenous to Central America, avocado, rich in vitamins A and C and other important nutrients, gives elasticity, tone, and smoothness to the hair.

Aloe vera, the elixir of life known for its rejuvenating powers and its healing and soothing properties, is another source for rehydration and soothing the scalp.

Apricot is rich in antioxidants flanked in vitamin E, it provides shine and softness, and protects color from fading.

Barley aids in nourishment without weighing down the strands. I like this for ultra fine and or oily hair.

Accompanied with hot steam from the mist of your shower, from the sauna at a spa, or a salon favorite, a mechanical steamer, this will impart optimum hydration.

Outside in the sun? Leave your conditioner in your hair and reap the benefits from this mighty resource!

In addition, herbs and minerals are especially helpful for irritated scalps. Helichrysum, which is native to Africa, has an astringent effect thanks to its calming properties.

Burdock "Herbarium Apulei" is another astringent used to restore natural balance to the scalp.

In addition to strengthening weak, fragile hair here are a few options.

Through my experience, I have found that rejuvenators with bamboo help produced new hair for clients suffering hair loss.

Basil is another strengthener, the origin of which is Africa and India. Legend holds that it contains valuable vitamins that strengthen the hair fibers.

Ginkgo biloba nicknamed "the Tree of Life," helps with micro-circulation, fortifying strength and vigor for growing hair.

Again, aloe vera seals in vibrant nutrients, nourishing and rehydrating the epidermis, and strengthening fibers from within.

You can see that conditioning the hair restructures fragile, overstressed hair and in some cases reverses balding and slows the aging process.

When your hair is weak and snaps, breaks, or sheds, it is generally deprived and needs a supplement infusion to heal it topically or internally. However, if the hair receives too much protein, it can have a polar affect and break the hair even more, or too much moisture will make it extremely soft and limp. Therefore, moderation is the key, to be on the safe side alternate one for the other every few treatments.

Restoring your hair with a nourishment treatment is equivalent to eating a balanced diet.

One of my favorites is NutriRich. It is a suitable conditioner for all hair types, infused with Brazil nut for nourishment and softness and Macadamia nut for protection and smoothness.

This formula is another part of my arsenal.

Supple Application:

Once you've found and chosen the conditioner that works in harmony with your hair, start kneading it with your hands, feeling the essence of the product binding to your hair. Start with a modest amount of balm; you can always apply more as needed.

You want to be mindful of waste, products infused with all this goodness for your hair's well-being come at a premium price. I prefer applying the balm with my fingers and the palms of my hands, because it warms the product and spreads it evenly throughout. At this point I am able to realize the distressed areas and feel the different textures in the hair, spotting the areas that require more or less attention.

Continue to direct the conditioner down the length of the hair, regardless of the texture, even if the hair is short. At this point the scales are absorbing the nutrients, penetrating and transforming your hair.

If your hair is straight, wavy, curly, or coiled, gliding down the length instead of using a circular motion enhances the sublime experience of watching your hair grow.

Remember the hairline (edges) around the entire circumference of your head. Repeat the same movement here. Later I speak a bit on cowlicks. There may be one here, so move in the direction you see your hair naturally falling. This will also protect your hairline and encourage growth.

I will repeat this until I'm out of breath… and I am. Include the hairline in the entire hair care routine. Two areas that are the most porous, neglected, and absolutely vulnerable are the hairline and the ends.

My preference is to start applying the product to the hairline first and then continue applying the product throughout the rest of the hair. In practicing, rarely have I seen a head of hair with only one texture throughout the entire head, so apply an extra dose of attention where you think it is needed.

The Spiral:

The golden spiral that connects us all to the universe, the cowlick.

A cowlick is a pattern in which hair grows in a directional circle.

Cowlicks usually occur at the crown near the top of the head; however, they can appear anywhere, including the hairline.

Be mindful of this when you're frustrated because it can be resistant and does not comply. This area also needs tender, loving attention.

Following the direction of the cowlick when applying your product will help alleviate that mysterious breakage "always in that one area!"

When you follow your hair's growth pattern, the improvement will be astonishing!

Go with the flow…

Once you've applied the reconstructor to your hair, this is now the best time to detangle your hair.

Detangling:

Using a large tooth comb, (never use a brush as your hair is now in its most vulnerable state) to distribute the conditioner through the hair, be very gentle, so as not to attack your hair.

Simplicity Isn't Easy… Take Time To Love On It.

Carefully comb through each strand of hair, starting at the ends and moving to the scalp.

As in the first step of the shampoo process, part the hair in sections of four, allowing the comb to glide though every strand to receive the benefits of the nutrients from the conditioner.

When in the shower, secure your hair on top of your head and intensify the treatment with steam or a plastic cap while you continue bathing. Once you are ready to rinse the conditioner, if possible use cool water to rinse the hair and scalp.

Adjusting the water temperature increases blood flow, decreases flakiness, soothes an irritated scalp, and nourishes the hair with what it needs while releasing what it doesn't. An extended benefit is that the water seals the cuticle, promoting a brilliant shine and better resilience!

That is what a cool water rinse can do for you!

At first the cool water may curl your toes but OMG it is so refreshing, and you will see immediate results also in your skin.

Now, what to do after the rinse?

Stress-less Hair:

Wrap the hair in a turban. this assists in absorbing excess water without disturbing the curl and prepares the hair for step three.

Why a turban?

The turban is achieved by using three corners of a towel to make a triangle, then using the fourth corner to overlap the triangle and tuck to absorb water from your hair.

Turbans assist in absorbing the water from the hair and scalp without disrupting the cuticle or your curls. This is an alternative to roughly drying the hair, which is like rubbing two sticks together trying to start a fire, causing friction and contributing to unnecessary breakage and frizz.

Visualize your hair in the towel drying it with the friction of the two sticks…

The turban prevents fraying and also helps sustain curls and waves when leaving the towel undisturbed, it also means less work drying your hair.

The hair air-dries in its natural state, thereby maximizing the texture you've been nourishing in steps one and two. It is ready to wear if you choose to go without heat. At this stage the curls have settled with optimum definition and plop!

My towel of choice is a cotton hand towel. Other materials, such as microfiber, are also good; this is equivalent to a t-shirt. Microfiber works well to retain water in the hair. However, I get consistent results with lightweight cotton.

This small towel constructs a tighter turban and quickly absorbs excess moisture, and reinforces a defined texture without having to use a diffuser if you choose. Of course, if you have mounds of hair, a larger towel is more useful. Although my young client Tiffani, who has mounds of hair, prefers to leave her hair sopping wet before starting her two-strand twist set. She doesn't use a towel at all.

Next question… should I use a leave-in conditioner, after already conditioning my hair?

Absolutely!

I cannot proceed without this step!

This final phase combats frizz, creates a barrier between moisture and air, and protects the hair from heat damage. This is an opportunity to seal the cuticle with another layer of botanicals provided by nature's healing powers.

If you want body and flow, this step is the way to go!

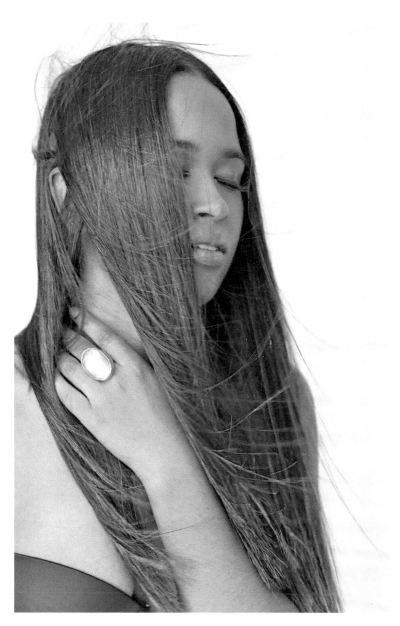

Hair speaks for you. Let's talk about it.

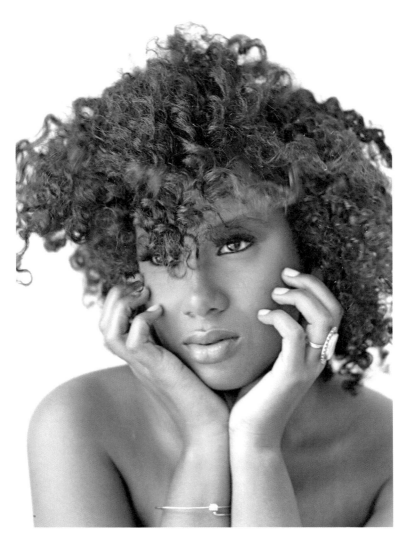

Natural curls bounce better when hydrated with a moisture
cocktail conditioner and intensified with a steamer.

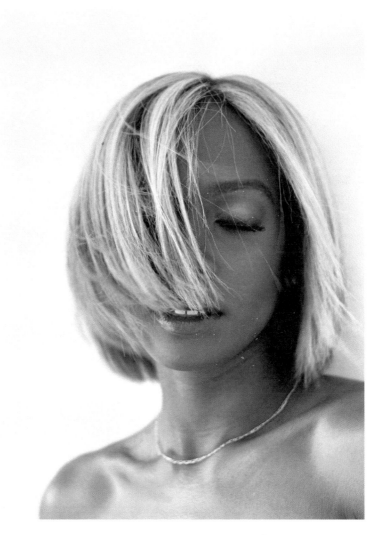

Protect color treated hair with shampoo formulated
to enhance and extend the intensity of the hue.

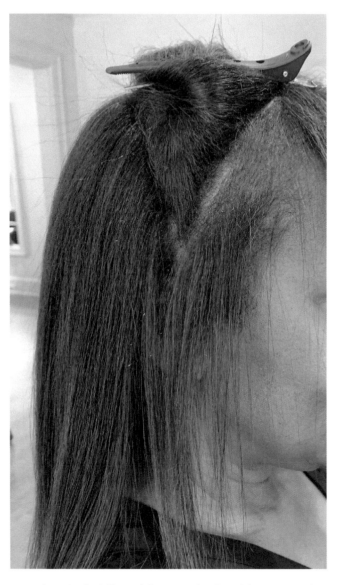

Stressing the hairline with excessive brushing, or neglect
causes the "edges" (hairline) to slowly disappear...
refrain from brushing, and see the hairline reappear.

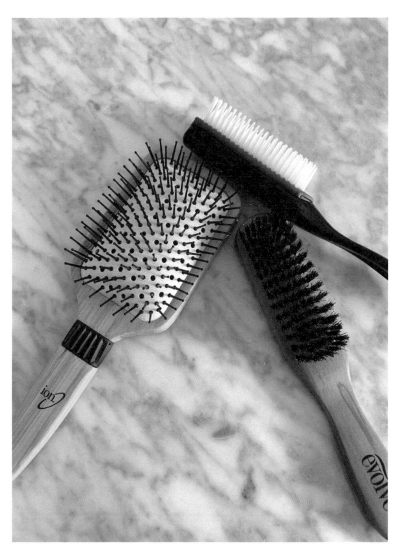

Brushes have a purpose;
however, used improperly
can destroy the hair.

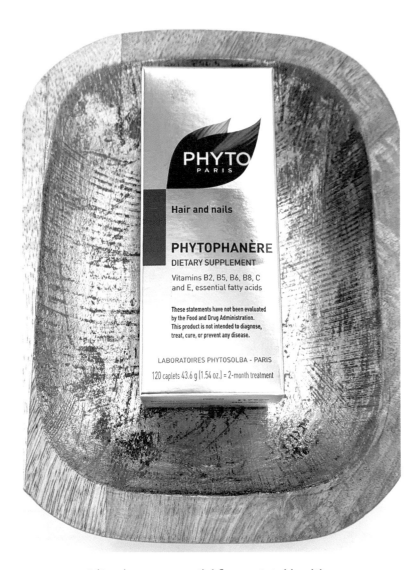

Vitamins are essential for our total health...
include a hair supplement to boost the hair's health.

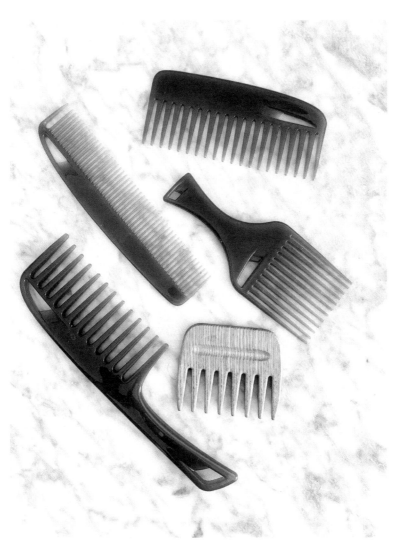

The hair can thrive when you use protective tools.

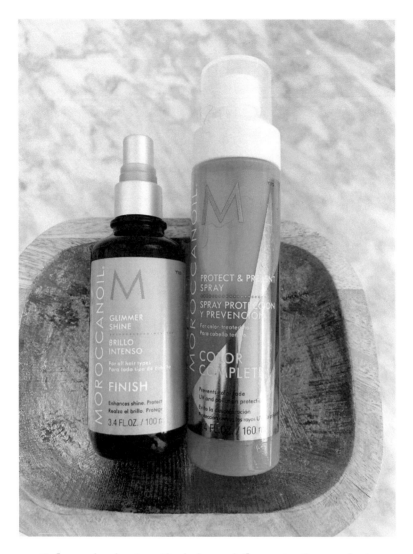

Before using heat on the hair reach for protective products
that shield the hair from heat damage.

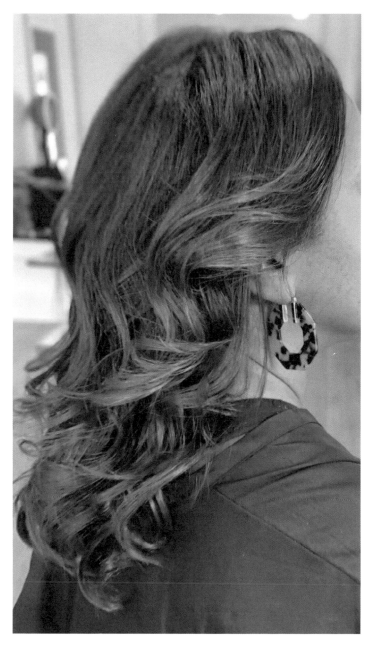

Results are rewarding when the client
and stylist work in tandem.

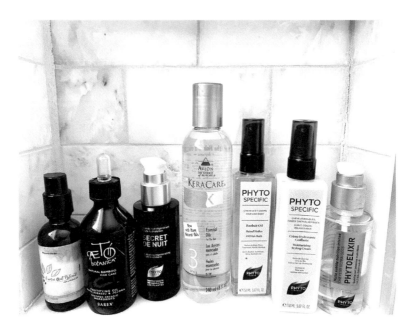

Oils are an ancient method for soothing dryness,
imparting shine, and healing the hair. Love in a bottle.

DETANGLING AGAIN

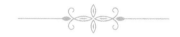

Ouch!

WARNING: abrasive and excessive combing produces unnecessary breakage—tread with caution and treat your hair gently…

Continue to practice patience, and if you stay with this technique, you will achieve your desired long-hair goal. Now that you're preparing your hair for combing after the first and second steps, remove the turban you've created to absorb the water. Once you have removed the turban, apply your leave-in cocktail.

I love to use a serum that adds shine and a fixative for memory. Barex has a line called Oliosetta that provides two restorative ingredients specifically for this purpose infused with linseed oil for strength and silk proteins. Neither my clients nor myself can live without it.

There are many choices for this portion of taking the Beast Out of Beauty. If you haven't already incorporated this in your routine, please do.

You will see and feel a significant difference. Even after many years, clients still query about how their hair lasts so long after their service. My answer is the leave-in conditioner; I can't live without a good one!

Next, if you desire to keep your curls or waves, refrain from over-combing with the comb or your fingers.

Combing excessively through your hair, even using your fingers, will disturb your curl pattern.

If you are finished at this step and you are wearing your hair in its natural glory or letting it air-dry, then apply your finishing product over the leave-in conditioner to complete your last step.

However, if you insist on using a comb to ensure each strand has received the product to lock in the curl, then comb very carefully and gingerly through each section.

Be it mousse, gel, or any cocktail you choose, continue to proceed with your finishing routine.

I think you will be quite happy with the integrity of your hair at this point.

Adding these simple but specific steps to your self-care regimen will help you to achieve your Long-Hair Goals in no time!

Implements:

Another familiar tip is using a wide- toothed comb for pre-venting excessive hair loss from tugging and tearing wet hair while detangling. One of my absolute favorite tools that glides through the hair is a keratin argan-infused comb. It is part of my secret arsenal for growing healthy hair.

Once, while practicing in the salon, I had a client who had a comb since forever, it seemed.

She didn't want to part with it to save her life. Finally, after much persuasion, Toni finally tried the same tool at home that I use at the salon. She saw a significant difference in the quality of her hair. Not only did she see her length remain on the ends, but also—what I was most excited about—her hairline returned!

Her original thoughts were that by using her favorite comb and feeling her hair pop and crackle she was detangling the snarls, making it better. Instead the complete opposite was occurring. The popping she heard was the sound of snap and breakage. Once she switched and used the argon-infused comb, she saw her hairline return and realized how much more hair she had!

The hairline, aka edges, need not be short and damaged, an island onto itself. The hairline is an integral part of the entire picture. This one small gesture of changing an implement used for grooming the hair made a world of difference, and Toni and I have since been a client-stylist team for quite a while.

In summary, if you need to separate your hair into sections, do so, take your time, and don't rush and rake through your hair. Give yourself enough time for your regimen so it won't become overwhelming. Refrain from forcing the comb through your tufts of hair, resulting in frayed strands. They will continue to unravel, and you'll never see the light of day when it comes to healthy ends.

Simplicity isn't easy, love on your hair...

FINISHING

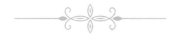

How can I get a salon-like finish at home?

Ready to wear your hair straight or just a simple blowout?

Here are a few tips to get you there:

Blow-drying is the most popular and quickest method to acquire a smooth luminous look.

Let's start with the artistry toward successfully achieving your flawless finish. We've already gone through three steps to get you to this point. Having already prepped your hair with a cocktail to effectively prevent heat damage, now we'll move on to the dryer.

The most frequently asked questions are…

Which tools are the best?

Should I use a brush or a comb or an attachment?

What kind of blow-dryer should I use?

Do I sit under the dryer before I blow-dry?

How do I use the nozzle that comes with the blow-dryer, and exactly what is it for?

Do I need to blow-dry at all?

Each approach presents a different type of finish from whichever method you choose to use.

From straight, slightly straight, to crinkle, this exercise is all about doing it with ease.

Start with choosing a blow-dryer with the latest technology.

A thermal, nano, or ionic blow-dryer ensures a smooth finish in half the drying time of the older appliances. Using the current models available with the latest technology will protect the hair and your nerves, and by the time this is published, a newer model will be on the market! However, with the convenience of the retail world at your fingertips, you can find this equipment at your nearest Ulta Beauty center, Sephora, Sally Beauty Supply or online.

The best advice is to consult your stylist when in doubt. They are most familiar with your hair and can tell you which appliance would best fit your needs and budget for superior results.

In comparison, I have found one brand may be suitable for fine fragile hair while another brand is best for thick, coarse hair.

The latest dryers enhance the hair with shine by respecting the cuticle and refrain from over-drying the hair. In choosing a dryer with the latest technological advancements in hair care, you won't regret the investment—it is well worth it.

The artistic technique I am sharing with you will help you effortlessly acquire a salon-like finish.

This will also rescue your hair and arms, prevent over-drying, and protect against unnecessary damage.

In addition, you can achieve smooth, luminous hair in half the time, and this step will prepare your hair for a flat iron, or curling iron if you prefer.

I hope these tips serve you well in keeping with the time you will save with modern technology and this fourth step.

Let's GO!

Start with guiding and gliding the blow-dryer in one direction down the length of the hair, preferably with the nozzle that came with the box, keeping in step with the same precautionary techniques we used in steps one two and three. This will remove the water from the hair quickly and efficiently while gently sealing the protective cocktail into the cuticle.

Move around the head clockwise, working the dryer from the roots all the way to the ends.

Do not stop along the mid-shaft (in the middle); flow with the dryer to the ends of the hair.

When blow-drying sporadically, drying the hair without any specific direction and allowing it to fly freely, the hair dries in a crinkled state, resulting in frizzy hair.

This is beautiful—that is, if this is your intended style—however, this is much more work and stressful if you want a smooth look.

I start with the speed on high with a nozzle adjacent to the width of the hair, blowing in one direction pushing the water away and out of the hair.

Consistently smooth the hair with the nozzle before applying the comb or brush to straighten it, consequently relieving the strands of any tugging while straightening.

Please take note there are many ways to achieve anything. I am only sharing my success with clients and my method for retaining the length over many years when using heat. When I approach drying the hair for a straight style, I prefer the high setting versus the low setting to start with, then using the cool setting at the very end.

It helps to ensure the hair is dry, eliminating reversion, especially on a humid day. I also prefer using a nozzle on the end of the dryer; you will definitely have more control of your hair during the drying process. Your results will pay off with a smoother cuticle, which will reflect more light and resist frizz and humidity with longer staying power for your finish.

Earlier, I stated there are different techniques for different results, and there isn't a wrong way. However, what I just shared works well for a smooth, salon-like blow-dry for all types and textures of hair.

When asked which tool is best for blow-drying, I suggest a heavy comb made by Black Diamond or DuPont. They have weight and retain some of the heat from the dryer, delivering smooth results. Having a standing advantage as the stylist, I use a paddle brush. It is efficient and quickly dries the hair.

If you prefer to use an attachment, again less stress to the hair is the end goal. Section in fours and start in the back where the hair is thickest. You tend to have more energy and patience when you start, so try beginning in the back in the occipital area where the hair is thickest.

Pause, then finish the front, where you have more patience and a better view of what's going on, then pull it all together with the final blow through. Frustration and weariness while doing your hair is another reason for predisposed breakage, so take your time. I find being in a hurry never turns out well, not even in the salon.

Now that you've completed step four, give yourself a break. Before you complete your final step with the flat or curling iron, grab a heat protector spray or serum to guard your strands and especially your ends from the flat iron.

Flat Iron:

Moderately apply this protection, too much isn't good because the hair becomes gummy and stiff, which make conditions ripe for cooking the hair. Which brings to mind, a frequently asked question, which temperature setting should you use when initially flat ironing fresh clean hair? Answer: the density of the hair will determine the setting.

I do prefer to start higher than lower. The reason being if you continue to repeat ironing the hair on a low setting, you have actually increased the amount of heat, and the possibility of scorching the hair. Proceed in sections, and within those sections use smaller sections. Using smaller sections may seem tedious; nevertheless, it decreases curling the same strand over and over again.

Getting the finish you want with the least amount of heat is the ultimate goal!

One and done achieving your desired look.

Congratulations!

Patience is a virtue when it comes to healthy hair…

BRUSHING

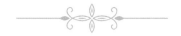

The good, the bad, and the ugly…

The benefit of brushing is that it feels oh so good on the scalp while stimulating the blood flow, which promotes growth, all while soothing the senses and encouraging relaxation in the process.

Brushing also removes dead skin cells, ushering oxygen to the epidermis for supreme airflow to the scalp.

And still leading the way to droopy eyes. The benefit of the 100-strokes-a-day rule is all that I have mentioned previously along with the distribution of the sebum (natural oils) from the scalp down the length and to the ends of the hair. This in turn provides natural hydration and protection for your strands.

This is the epitome of using what God gave you to enhance your natural beauty. However, when the brush is used aggressively it becomes a weapon, trying to tame the hair instead of loving on it, and this is what inevitably happens….

In my 30-plus years of practicing and diagnosing hair problems, I find brushing textured hair has been the catalyst to mysterious breakage. During consultations with new clients and discussing their hair loss concerns, I have learned that the most common problem has been improper brushing.

For generations, the timeless dialogue for growing long, beautiful hair has been "give your hair 100 strokes a day and the hair will grow long and strong."

Only when it is done at a snail's pace, ever so slowly, and the scales aren't compromised does this practice has its rewards.

With the brush, start gliding at the scalp area where the sebum is; the hair is strongest at the root area, through the mid-shaft also known as the middle, and then the most fragile at the oldest part of the hair, the ends. The brush distributes the oils throughout the hair. Be mindful when brushing textured hair harshly—it disturbs the imbrications. The scales become frayed, sparse, and dull, and frizzy strands are indicative of unwanted breakage.

In cases where there are delicate areas around the hairline, the repeated intense striking of the scalp with the brush can cause irreversible damage, initiating possible hair loss. Children are especially vulnerable along with too tight ponytails. Sadly, by young adulthood, their hairline is completely gone. Imagine brushing your face as often and as aggressively as you brush your hair.

What would occur? Your face would probably suffer from scarring, perhaps severe scarring.

Raking the brush hurriedly through your hair daily compromises the potential for substantial length.

I simply tell my clients to stop brushing.

STOP the BRUshInG!

The frowns appear, and denial sets in, but the evidence is there, and I can always tell when they have done so. Once they refrain from this ritual, they see immediate results, especially around the edges!

While proper brushing stimulates blood flow, improper brushing can strip the hair of its life, luster, and potential length. The general question that follows is "Will my hair ever come back?"

With intense treatments and frequent trims, the hair may recover in time.

Realize that your strands are delicate fibers comparable to silk that fray and tear very easily when handled improperly. By now, I may sound like a broken record, but I can't stress enough how damaging, improper manipulation affects your hair. Doing this daily, whether it is you, your mom, and especially your grandmother, you are doing your crown and glory a disservice.

Don't attack it!

Love on it…

Mind you, I am speaking of unconscious brushing; however, when my clients stop altogether, they do see immediate results. They are amazed how this simple habit has robbed their hair. However, if you cannot do without your brush, let's take a look at the best brush for your hair care needs.

The best brush for the 100 strokes a day is one with natural boar hairs. This should be done gently and methodically, literally like a sloth climbing a tree. The bristles from the boar hairs capture the sebum from your scalp, and as you glide the brush down the length of the hair, the oil is then redistributed upon the shaft, whereupon the hair is conditioned naturally.

Remember to follow through to the very ends and not flicker the brush briskly, contributing to splitting and compromising your length. A Denman brush is used to lift the hair and glide through and create body. It is effective for hair that is flat or lies close to the scalp.

This brush is a classic and is often used when blow-drying. A round brush is also used for this purpose, creating mounds of body and volume when drying the hair. Then there is everyone's favorite, the paddle brush, great for blowouts, gathering the hair and streaming in unison with the dryer, creating a straight finish.

At the end of the day, brushes aren't all bad—they do serve a purpose, and it is how you use them that makes the difference.

Just keep it simple, and remember: less is more!

VITAMINS, NUTRITION, *and* ESSENTIAL OILS

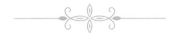

Your hair is a filter…
How to keep your hair young?
The papilla is the nexus for healthy hair!
What is this, you ask?

The papilla are cells below the epidermis supplied with nutrients from the blood and lymph system nourishing the hair follicle, enriching a healthy head of hair. When this system is compromised, and the blood supply is depleted of essential nutrients—A for the cells, B for biotin, C and E for antioxidants, iron, zinc, and protein—hair will cease to flourish, get thinner, break off, and appear to stop growing, therefore looking old.

Your hair is a filter…

The symmetry of nutrients keeps our organs functioning properly. The same applies for our hair, skin, and nails. What we choose to consume and life's experiences have a cause and effect on how our body functions and inevitably the fate of our strands.

Let's say you were to spoon-feed your hair daily, well, the hair's vital nutrient of choice would be blood. Yes, juicy vitamin A, B, C, and E enriched blood, enhanced by eating broccoli, kale, collards, beets, spinach, and other vitamin-enriched vegetables that also serve as antioxidants.

Live foods are an excellent source for nourishing blood cells that fuel the bulb, which in turn fuels the follicle and promotes a healthy, flesh-colored scalp that is the root of healthy hair.

Grandma was right! "You are what you eat."

Consider cleansing your body, detoxifying and rebooting your system altogether.

Unhealthy eating and illness will propel your system into over-drive protecting the organs first, and when this occurs, the hair suffers from nutrient depletion. This is the reason the hair starts to shed when the body is in distress or going through physical changes.

Another path to healthy hair is heaven-sent aqua. Water cleanses and purifies and is the ultimate life source. The daily intake flushes the system free of toxins and hydrates your skin and fibrous strands. The intake of pollutants, such as smoking, medications, and other foreign substances dehydrates the body, leading to dull, brittle, weak hair that is slow to grow, another component of thinning. Nourish the blood and the hair will thrive long and strong.

In addition, phytonutrients are amazing purifiers to help this along; vegetables and berries, citrus fruits, and melons such as, red and yellow peppers, sweet potatoes, and antioxidant foods rich in color curtail inflammation at the root and promote healthy, functional cells.

Enriching your system is not only beneficial for your hair but also for your skin and your organs; your entire body will salute you!

Juicing and organic juice are nutritious ways to digest a meal on the go and to receive the nutrients of a full meal. Multivitamins are another good source to supplement your diet.

They are full of B vitamins, which are vital for hair growth and a great source of energy.

Food grown today can sometimes be a mystery, deprived of the earth's nutrients and sprinkled with chemicals to encourage expedient growth.

Digesting a vitamin supplement daily or as often as possible can offset the negative effects and protect the body at the same time, a twofer!

A, a natural fat, is vital for our scalp and for all our organs to function properly. B-Complexes, B12 and biotin, stimulate our hair growth and provides energy when we are feeling sluggish. C ensures a healthy immune system. Darling D wards off disease and viruses and E protects our follicles. Zinc ensures the absorption of all nutrients—all of these are found in a multivitamin. The Centrum brand is tried and true and covers the entire vitamin alphabet. It has worked for me and many of my clients without fail through the years. Combine it with a vitamin specifically for hair growth and, voilà! Your garden will continue to grow!

Another one of my faves is Phytophanere. I have used and suggested this vitamin for my entire career. It is by far the best vitamin for hair restoration I have ever used! I have witnessed 99 percent positive results when it is taken daily, even when a dermatologist has diagnosed alopecia aerate.

I have seen hope grow from this little glass bottle!

In order to give your hair its best chance at looking, being, and staying young and healthy, try eating a new food with nutrients enriched with B6, B12, E, and beyond. In essence, your hair is a filter and the evidence of your lifestyle flows through your hair.

Laughter and exercise relieve stress and facilitate oxygen and blood flow to your crown, enriching your glory! The hair tells no lies. Love on yourself and your hair will mirror just that…

Start to incorporate and indulge in the healthy fats found in fish and natural oils. Cook with olive oil, eat wild caught salmon or sushi, or take it in the form of a supplement such as cod liver oil in conjunction with applying oil to your hair externally to increase your shine!

Healthy fat is another little secret in producing sebum, another variable in the equation of looking good. Every morning I take and suggest to my clients Norwegian lemon-flavored cod liver oil; a teaspoon daily keeps the heebie-jeebies away. I find that not only does my oh so dry hair respond to it; my joints and limbs are agile and limber.

And for me and my family, it's the go-to when the sniffles want to creep up! Start with small baby steps if this is all new to you. Although I have to say, you will see some things change for the better if you give it a try.

Oil or not to oil?

As for applying oils to the hair and scalp, if it feels good and relieves and soothes the scalp, go for it!

In the past, I didn't care for artificial oil on the scalp, but with the accessibility to a variety of botanicals, this makes for a holistic experience. Curlier or too coarse hair needs assistance with hydrating curls. So, there is a need to dress and apply oil throughout the hair for increasing nourishment and shine.

MOROCCAN OIL is a very popular brand, formulated with its infamous argan oil and known for its regenerating and protective properties. It is a favorite for all hair types. Another favorite is Kera Care Essential Oil. It's infused with a plethora of essential botanicals. They include sunflower seed, which is rich in minerals and protects color-treated hair from oxidation, peanut oil, which is high in vitamin E, warding off free radicals. Included also is aloe barbadensis leaf extract, known as the elixir of life, sweet almond oil, a moisturizer, and a familiar favorite, castor oil, just to name a few of these therapeutic oils and their natural benefits.

I use a variety of oils regularly on clients; these ancient elixirs have their own distinct character, each nourishing and healing with the purpose they were meant for. Oils have been a cure-all for me since I was very young. They have been my remedy for my oh so dry skin to my extremely dry hair. I know which light to heavy formula works for any season and region.

From the healing of baobab oil by Phyto to the protection and shine of Moroccan oil formulas, botanicals nourish the essence of our being. Each chapter covered here requires something different. a little less a little more... I hope these few tips will find you well and enhance your self-care ritual. Remember, simply love on your hair.

Being fabulous isn't easy...

PSYCHOLOGY

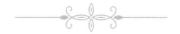

Hair is powerful…

Hair is the first feature we adjust when our lives change.

It's the first feature people see and describe after you encounter or meet someone for the first time.

Question: "How are they wearing their hair?"

The conversation about hair is ancient. Healthy hair personifies vitality and sensuality for everyone. It is seductive. Hair can reflect our confidence and our self-esteem.

Researching our origins and our ancestry helps us realize how our textures materialized.

In many cultures it is part of a religious practice, when we alter our lives cutting our hair is a form of spiritual healing, starting anew.

The way we feel about ourselves living in confidence, attractiveness, admiration—is mired in our connective feelings with our hair.

Hair reigns supreme. Influencers today continue to set the trends with how society reacts to new and different hairstyles.

Hair has always been the topic of discussion that is then dissected and copied.

The old adage that your hair is your glory is true. When it is freshly cut and coiffed, women and men alike have more stride in their glide, or may I say, more swag. Hair personifies health, beauty, and affluence and is admired by all.

Historically and presently, it is associated with status. Let me just say an undetectable hair weave or lace front worn by some is not cheap. Your image personified by your hair invokes a story about you, whether you realize it or not, through the style you choose to wear.

Suggestively wearing your hair in a neat and tight style suggests you are conservative, reserved, and all about business. Natural or color-treated blondes give an image of light and delight. They are a joy to have around, hence the phrase "blondes have more fun!" Redheads were known for their fiery tempers—don't cross them, or there would be hell to pay. A short, cropped haircut suggests you are creative and progressive, suggesting the artsy, modern-type.

These images and classifications mold a psychological subliminal influence when creating characters for movies the theatre and such. The conversation continues, as we are waiting for The Crown Act to pass in the Senate. Signing legislature abolishing a law prohibiting women of color from wearing their hair freely through out all of the 50 states. This is still part of the kitchen conversation. Hair is p-o-w-e-r-f-u-l.

Finale…LOVE ON YOUR HAIR!

ACKNOWLEDGMENTS

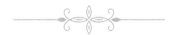

This project is to leave you with a few tips to enhance your regiment producing a healthy head of beautiful hair. I say, "Simplicity isn't easy" often because we often think "Just one more thing." then we over shoot our hair goal. I hope these few pages take some of The Beast Out of Beauty and contributes to growing your hair strong, healthy and as long, or sassy as you desire.

I would like to acknowledge my loving family Marsalis, my son, Elwood & Virgie my parents, James my husband and my brother Anthony for their endless love. Cynthia Craig, Triba Gary, Lori Wilson, Linda Clark and the Richardson's for guiding me through this project.

The loyal, brilliant U salon family and clients, who through the years have become dear to my heart-Thank you for entrusting me with your crowns of glory sprinkled with encouragement, wisdom and laughter.

Love you, to be continued…

RESOURCES

Barex Italiana

Aveda Institute, Cosmetology Curriculum

Joc

A New World Of Haircare

Phtyo Paris Training Manual

Phyto Specific Training Manual

MOROCCANOIL Product Guide

Marie Claire Magazine 2017

Beauty Lauchpad 2020

.